I0841817

THE CANDIDA CURE FOR WOMEN

Unveiling the Candida Cure, Empowering Women's Health

STEVE OPERA

Copyright © 2023

All Rights Are Reserved

The content in this book may not be reproduced, duplicated, or transferred without the express written permission of the author or publisher. Under no circumstances will the publisher or author be held liable or legally responsible for any losses, expenditures, or damages incurred directly or indirectly as a consequence of the information included in this book.

Legal Remarks

Copyright protection applies to this publication. It is only intended for personal use. No piece of this work may be modified, distributed, sold, quoted, or paraphrased without the author's or publisher's consent.

Disclaimer Statement

Please keep in mind that the contents of this booklet are meant for educational and recreational purposes. Every effort has been made to offer accurate, up-to-date, reliable, and thorough information. There are, however, no stated or implied assurances of any kind. Readers understand that the author is providing competent counsel. The content in this book originates from several sources. Please seek the opinion of a competent professional before using any of the tactics outlined in this book. By reading this book, the reader agrees that the author will not be held accountable for any direct or indirect damages resulting from the use of the information contained therein, including, but not limited to, errors, omissions, or inaccuracies.

TABLE OF CONTENTS

INTRODUCTION

In a society where fitness and health are our top priorities, Candida is a silent killer that frequently goes unnoticed and wrecks havoc on women's lives. "The Candida Cure for Women" is a powerful source of empowerment and hope for those dealing with this common but frequently misdiagnosed illness.

You will set out on a life-changing adventure through the pages of this extensive guide, one that reveals the complexities of Candida overgrowth and equips you with the information and resources necessary to overcome it. Naturally occurring yeast in the body called Candida becomes a powerful enemy when it multiplies unchecked, causing a host of symptoms that interfere with day-to-day functioning.

This best-selling book provides a definitive plan curated by professionals that combines the most recent scientific knowledge with doable, practical steps—it's not simply another flimsy promise of relief. This book will help you combat Candida head-on by providing you with comprehensive diagnosis, treatment, and long-term management options, as well as by shedding light on the mysterious disease.

With great care, each chapter is designed to lead you through the maze of symptoms, triggers, and solutions. You'll delve into the world of natural medicines, examine the subtleties of dietary changes, and adopt lifestyle adjustments that give you back control over your health. Moreover, it offers priceless guidance on managing the psychological and emotional aspects of having Candida.

This is a life raft in the choppy waters of Candida overgrowth, not just a book. "The Candida Cure for Women" is a lifeline for anyone suffering from persistent symptoms or hearing the first murmurs of Candida. It promotes understanding, empowerment, and, in the end, freedom from the disease's clutches.

Prepare to set off on a path of self-exploration, recovery, and vitality restoration. Together, let's reveal the way to live a life free from Candida's darkness and welcome the brightness of holistic health.

You are welcome to modify this introduction to fit the exact message and tone you wish to convey about the book!

CHAPTER ONE

UNDERSTANDING CANDIDA

What is Candida?

Candida is a form of yeast or fungus that is found in trace amounts in the human body naturally, mostly in the skin, mucous membranes, and digestive tract. Most of the time, Candida coexists with other microbes innocuously and causes no problems. It can, however, overgrow in some circumstances and cause a number of health issues.

Candida Species: There are other species of Candida, but Candida albicans is the one that affects people most frequently. Other species, each with distinct traits and susceptibilities, such as Candida glabrata, Candida tropicalis, Candida krusei, and Candida auris, can also cause infections.

Candida Overgrowth Causes:

1. Antibiotics and Medications: Antibiotics have the ability to upset the body's bacterial equilibrium, which promotes the growth of Candida.

2. Weakened Immune System: People with weakened immune systems are more vulnerable to Candida overgrowth.

3. High-Sugar Diets: Consuming too much sugar might nourish Candida and encourage its growth.

4. Hormonal Changes: Candida growth can be exacerbated by hormonal shifts, which can occur during pregnancy or while taking birth control medications.

5. Stress and Bad Lifestyle Choices: Stress impairs immunity, increasing the body's vulnerability to Candida infections.

Conditions Resulting from Overgrowth of Candida:

1. Oral Thrush: A covering of white, cottage cheese-like substance on the inner cheeks and tongue.

2. Yeast Infections of the Vagina: Typical signs and symptoms include burning, itching, and strange discharge in the vaginal region.

3. Skin Infections: Warm, moist skin areas, such as those under the breasts or in skin folds, can develop red, itchy rashes due to Candida.

4. Digestive Issues: Gas, bloating, diarrhea, and constipation are some of the symptoms that can result from an overgrowth in the gut.

5. Systemic Candidiasis: Candida can enter the bloodstream and cause potentially fatal systemic infections in extreme cases or in immunocompromised people.

Causes and Triggers

Of course! Overgrowth of Candida can be brought on by a number of circumstances. These are a few typical reasons and catalysts:

1. Use of Antibiotics:

Although antibiotics are meant to eradicate dangerous germs, they can also upset the body's delicate balance of good bacteria. An environment conducive to Candida growth is produced by this imbalance.

2. Diets High in Carbohydrates and Sugar:

Sugar and processed carbs are Candida's main food sources. A diet rich in these nutrients may encourage the growth of Candida, leading to an overabundance of the fungus in the body.

3. Weakened Immune System: People who suffer from diseases like HIV/AIDS or disorders that require the use of immune-suppressive drugs are more vulnerable to Candida overgrowth.

4. Changes in Hormones:

Hormone fluctuations, such as those that occur during pregnancy, menstruation, or while taking birth control pills, might foster the growth of Candida.

5. Lifestyle and Stress Factors:

Prolonged stress impairs immunity, reducing the body's ability to fight off illnesses. Unhealthy lifestyle choices, such as sleeping too little or drinking too much alcohol, can also lead to Candida overgrowth.

6. Basis Medical Conditions:

Certain medical problems, such as autoimmune illnesses or diabetes, can foster an environment that is conducive to the growth of Candida. Diabetes causes high blood sugar, which is perfect for Candida growth, especially when it is not properly managed.

7. Climatic Variables:

Candida overgrowth can also result from prolonged exposure to moist or humid conditions, such as living in moldy surroundings or wearing wet clothes.

8. Immune System Weakness:

Unbalances in the gut microbiota brought on by things like a bad diet, frequent antacid use, or digestive problems might foster an environment that is favorable to Candida growth.

Candida Symptoms in Women

Of course! Women who have an overgrowth of Candida may have a range of symptoms. It's crucial to remember that each person will experience symptoms differently, and others may have few or none at all. The following are typical signs of female Candida overgrowth:

1. Yeast Infection of the Vagina:

- **Irritation and Itching:** Severe itching in and around the vaginal region is a typical symptom.
- **Abnormal Discharge:** There may be a thick, white discharge that resembles cottage cheese.
- **Burning Sensation:** Uncomfortable feeling or burning sensation, particularly after sexual activity or urine.

2. Oral Thrush:

- **White Patches:** Creamy white lesions on the roof of the mouth, inner cheeks, or tongue.
- **Soreness:** pain or discomfort in the throat or mouth.

3. Nail and Skin Infections:

- **Rash:** Red, swollen, or irritated skin, particularly in moist, warm places like the folds beneath the breasts.
- **Nail Changes:** Breakage, discoloration, or infection of the nails

4. Digestive Issues:

- **Bloating:** Experiencing gas or bloating after eating.
- **Digestive discomfort:** Constipation or diarrhea are examples of digestive discomfort.
- **Dietary Sensitivities:** heightened susceptibility to specific foods or intolerances

5. Mood swings and fatigue:

- **Fatigue:** Excessive tiredness or sluggishness, even after getting enough sleep.

- **Mood Swings:** shifts in mood, such as irritation or nervousness.

6. Recurrent UTIs (Urinary Tract Infections):

Frequent UTIs: Increased frequency of UTI bouts.

7. Dysregulations in the Menstrual Cycle:

Modifications in the Menstrual Flow: Disturbances in the cycling of the menstrual cycle.

8. Everlasting Yeast Infections:

Recurrent Recurrence: Getting infected with yeast more than once in a year.

9. In rare and severe cases, systemic symptoms:

Fever, chills, and possibly fatal consequences are possible signs in extreme cases of Candida overgrowth, where the infection becomes systemic. Systemic candidiasis, on the other hand, is less frequent and usually affects people with impaired immune systems.

CHAPTER TWO

DIAGNOSIS AND TESTING

Recognizing Candida Overgrowth

Identifying Candida overgrowth entails looking for physical signs as well as possible risk factors. Here's how you could identify it:

1. Oral thrush: which manifests as white patches in the mouth, tongue, or throat.

2. Genital Symptoms: persistent yeast infections, strange discharge, or vaginal irritation.

3. Skin Concerns: Red, scratchy rashes, particularly in regions that are warm and damp on the skin.

4. Digestive Issues: Constipation, diarrhea, gas, or bloating

5. Fatigue: having enough sleep yet still feeling worn out or lethargic.

6. Mood Changes: Anxiety, irritability, or mood swings without a clear explanation

7. Symptoms of the Urinary Tract: Chronic pain or infections of the urinary tract

Risk Factors:

1. Antibiotic Use: Frequent or recent use of antibiotics, upsetting the bacteria's normal equilibrium.

2. Dietary Factors: Consumption of alcohol, refined carbs, or high sugar intake

3. Immune System Weakness: The immune system is weakened by diseases including diabetes, autoimmune disorders, and HIV/AIDS, which increases the likelihood of Candida overgrowth.

4. Hormonal Changes: Pregnancy, birth control pills, or hormonal therapy

5. Chronic stress: Prolonged stress results in weakened immunity.

6. Previous Infections: A history of persistent candidiasis or yeast infections

Living or working in moist, moldy conditions constitutes the seventh type of environmental exposure.

Self-Assessment Tools: A few online or in-health resources are self-assessment tools, tests, or symptom checklists. They can be a preliminary sign of possible Candida overgrowth, but any concerns should be verified by a medical practitioner.

Medical Diagnosis: Evaluation of symptoms, physical examination, and occasionally laboratory testing are used to provide a diagnosis. Swabs, cultures, blood tests, or stool analysis may be performed by a medical professional to confirm the presence of Candida overgrowth, particularly in cases where symptoms are severe or persistent.

Medical Tests and Examinations

Of course! The diagnosis of Candida overgrowth or associated illnesses is made using a variety of medical tests and exams. Here are a few typical ones:

1. Physical Examination: A medical professional may perform a visual examination to look for vaginal symptoms connected to Candida overgrowth, skin rashes, or indications of mouth thrush.

2. Swab Tests:

Oral Swab: Using a mouth swab to identify oral thrush

Vaginal Swab: Taking a sample from the vaginal region in order to identify infections caused by yeast

3. Cultures and Microscopic Examination:

Culture Test: To determine the particular strain of Candida, a sample (swab, blood, urine, or other body fluids) is cultivated in a lab.

Microscope Analysis: Samples are examined under a microscope to check for the presence of Candida organisms.

4. Antibody Tests:

Blood Tests: Identifying antibodies the immune system produces against Candida.

Antigen Tests: Determining the presence of particular blood-borne Candida antigens

5. Stool Tests: Examining stool samples to find evidence of gastrointestinal system Candida overgrowth

6. Polymerase Chain Reaction (PCR) Testing: A molecular biology method for amplifying and identifying particular DNA sequences of Candida organisms.

7. Comprehensive Digestive Stool Analysis (CDSA): This test looks at a variety of stool components, including fungi, bacteria, and other gastrointestinal tract organisms that are both useful and dangerous.

8. Imaging Studies (Rarely performed): Imaging studies such as CT scans or MRIs may be performed to detect organ involvement in severe cases or when the Candida infection progresses.

Self-Assessment Tools

Self-assessment methods are helpful for people to determine whether they may have an overgrowth of Candida. It's crucial to remember that these instruments are just meant to serve as initial indicators and cannot replace expert medical guidance. The following self-assessment instruments are frequently used to determine whether Candida overgrowth is likely:

1. Questionnaires:

Yeast Infection Questionnaires: These inquire about complaints of the skin, mouth, or vaginal areas.

Symptom Questionnaires for Candida: Examine a variety of symptoms linked to Candida overgrowth, including skin disorders, exhaustion, and digestive troubles.

2. Online Assessments: A plethora of websites provide online checklists or quizzes aimed at assisting people in recognizing symptoms that may indicate a Candida problem.

3. Dietary Diaries: Monitoring dietary patterns, especially sugar intake, with a food journal can reveal hidden causes for Candida overgrowth.

4. Symptom Tracking Apps: These apps for smartphones let users monitor their symptoms over time, which can be used to find trends or connections between particular symptoms and possible triggers.

5. Test Kits for Home Use There are kits on the market that promise to identify Candida overgrowth. Stool tests and self-collection swabs are examples of this; however, their precision may differ.

Advice for Using Self-Assessment Tools:

Take into Account Several Symptoms: Candida overgrowth can show up in a number of different ways. Examine a variety of symptoms, not just one or two, to provide a more thorough assessment.

Ask for Professional Advice: Self-assessment tools are useful, but getting a good diagnosis and receiving the right therapy depend on seeing a healthcare provider.

Avoid Making Hasty Diagnoses: Overgrowth of Candida symptoms can mimic those of other illnesses. Refrain from self-diagnosing based just on web resources.

CHAPTER THREE

DIETARY STRATEGIES
Anti-Candida Diet Basics

Of course! Ten essential guidelines for an anti-Candida diet are as follows:

1. Reduce Sugar Intake:

Avoid Refined Sugars: Steer clear of refined sugars that can promote Candida growth, such as high-fructose corn syrup and white sugar.

Reduce Natural Sugars: Initially, cut back on high-sugar fruits and instead concentrate on low-sugar ones, such as berries.

2. Avoid high-carbohydrate foods: Limit Grains: Cut back on or completely avoid refined grains and foods that contain gluten, such as rye, wheat, and barley.

Observe Starches: Reduce your intake of starchy veggies like potatoes and increase your intake of low-starch options like leafy greens, broccoli, and cauliflower.

3. Support Non-Starchy Vegetables:

Go Eco-Friendly: Add an abundance of non-starchy, high-nutrient veggies, such as Brussels sprouts, zucchini, spinach, and kale.

4. Select Healthy Fats:

Healthy Oils: Make use of fats that reduce inflammation, such as avocado, coconut, and olive oils.

Omega-3s: Include foods high in omega-3 fatty acids, such as fatty fish, chia seeds, and flaxseeds.

5. Include High-Quality Protein Sources:

Lean Proteins: Choose fish, poultry, lean meats, and plant-based proteins such as tofu and lentils.

Red Meat Limit: When consuming, go for organic or grass-fed products and limit your intake.

6. Foods High in Probiotics:

Foods Fermented: Consume foods high in probiotics, such as kimchi, kefir, sauerkraut, and unsweetened yogurt, to help maintain a healthy gut microbiome.

7. Herbs and Spices:

Properties Against Fungi: Add herbs and spices like garlic, oregano, cinnamon, and turmeric that are known to have antifungal effects.

8. Aqueous:

Make Sure to Hydrate Well: To assist with detoxification and general wellness, drink plenty of water.

9. Steer clear of processed foods: Avoid processed foods. Get rid of packaged and processed foods that have artificial substances, preservatives, and additives.

10. Conscious Eating:

Consciously Eat: Eat with awareness, observing your body's signals of hunger and the effects of various foods.

Foods to Avoid and Embrace

Absolutely! Here are lists of foods to avoid and foods to embrace while on an anti-Candida diet:

Foods to Avoid:

1. Sugar and Sweeteners: White sugar, brown sugar, high-fructose corn syrup, maple syrup, honey, and artificial sweeteners.

2. High-Carb Foods: Refined grains (white bread, pasta), baked goods, cereals, and processed snacks.

3. Starchy Vegetables: Potatoes, yams, corn, and other high-starch root vegetables.

4. Fruits High in Sugar: Bananas, grapes, mangoes, and dried fruits with high sugar content.

5. Dairy Products: Cow's milk, cheeses, and sweetened yogurts (unless they contain live cultures without added sugars).

6. Processed and Junk Foods: fast food, processed meats, chips, and heavily processed snacks

7. Alcohol: Beer: Wine, and spirits can promote yeast growth and disrupt gut flora.

8. Condiments and Sauces: Ketchup, barbecue sauce, soy sauce (unless tamari), and commercially prepared dressings with added sugars

9. Caffeine and Stimulants: Coffee, black tea, energy drinks, and excessive caffeine-containing beverages.

10. Highly Processed Fats and Oils: Trans fats, hydrogenated oils, and refined vegetable oils like soybean or corn oil

Foods to Embrace:

1. Non-Starchy Vegetables:

leafy greens, broccoli, cauliflower, asparagus, bell peppers, and cucumbers.

2. Lean Proteins: Chicken, turkey, fish, eggs, tofu, legumes (in moderation), and plant-based protein sources.

3. Healthy Fats: Avocado, coconut oil, olive oil, flaxseeds, chia seeds, and nuts in moderation (like almonds and walnuts)

4. Low-Sugar Fruits: Berries (like blueberries, strawberries, and raspberries), green apples, and citrus fruits in moderation

5. Probiotic-Rich Foods: Unsweetened yogurt, kefir, sauerkraut, kimchi, and other fermented foods.

6. Herbs and Spices: Garlic, oregano, turmeric, ginger, cinnamon, and other spices with known antifungal properties.

7. Non-Caffeinated Beverages: Herbal teas, green tea, and plenty of water to stay hydrated.

8. Gluten-Free Grains: Quinoa, buckwheat, millet, and brown rice in moderation

9. Low-Sugar Sweeteners (in Moderation): Stevia or monk fruit as alternatives to sugar, in limited quantities

10. Nutrient-Dense Foods:

Focus on whole, unprocessed foods rich in vitamins, minerals, and antioxidants.

Meal Plans and Recipes

Creating meal plans for an anti-Candida diet involves focusing on whole, nutrient-dense foods while avoiding sugars, refined carbohydrates, and processed items. Here's a sample meal plan along with recipe ideas:

Sample Meal Plan:

Breakfast:

Chia Seed Pudding: Mix chia seeds with unsweetened almond milk, top with berries, and sprinkle with cinnamon.

Herbal Tea: Enjoy a cup of herbal tea.

Snack:

Cucumber Slices with Hummus: Use homemade hummus (chickpeas, garlic, lemon juice, and olive oil).

Lunch:

Grilled Chicken Salad: Grilled chicken breast on a bed of mixed greens, cucumbers, tomatoes, and a drizzle of olive oil and lemon juice

Quinoa (optional): A small portion of cooked quinoa on the side.

Snack:

Mixed Nuts: A handful of almonds, walnuts, and pumpkin seeds

Dinner:

Baked Salmon: Baked salmon fillet seasoned with herbs and lemon

Steamed Broccoli and Cauliflower: Served with a touch of olive oil and garlic.

Stir-Fried Greens: Sautéed spinach, kale, and Swiss chard with garlic and olive oil.

Recipe Ideas:

1. Cauliflower Rice Stir-Fry:

Ingredients: cauliflower rice, mixed vegetables, tofu or chicken, garlic, ginger, and tamari sauce.

Instructions: Sauté garlic and ginger, add vegetables and protein, and stir in cauliflower rice and tamari sauce.

2. Coconut Curry Chicken:

Ingredients: chicken breast, coconut milk, curry paste, onions, bell peppers, and spinach.

Instructions: Sauté onions, add chicken, then bell peppers, coconut milk, curry paste, and spinach; simmer until chicken is cooked.

3. Avocado and Tuna Salad:

Ingredients: canned tuna, avocado, mixed greens, cherry tomatoes, cucumber, olive oil, and lemon juice.

Instructions: Mix tuna with diced avocado, serve on a bed of greens, tomatoes, and cucumber, and dress with olive oil and lemon juice.

4. Roasted Vegetables:

Ingredients: Assorted vegetables (zucchini, bell peppers, carrots), olive oil, garlic, and herbs.

Instructions: Toss vegetables with olive oil, garlic, and herbs; roast in the oven until tender.

CHAPTER FOUR

LIFESTYLE CHANGES

Managing Stress and Candida

Stress does have an effect on Candida overgrowth because it compromises the immune system and interferes with the body's capacity to keep a healthy balance of microbes. One of the most important parts of managing Candida is managing stress. The following techniques can be used to reduce stress when treating Candida:

1. Stress Reduction Techniques: Mindfulness and Meditation: To quiet the mind and lower stress levels, engage in mindfulness exercises or meditation.

Deep Breathing: Practice yoga or deep breathing techniques to help you relax.

Progressive Muscle Relaxation: To relieve physical tension, tense and relax various muscle groups.

2. Regular Exercise: Take part in any kind of exercise you love, such as yoga, swimming, walking, or any regular physical activity. Exercise boosts the immune system and lowers stress.

3. Healthy Sleep Habits: Establish a calming bedtime routine and stick to a regular sleep schedule to ensure you get enough sleep.

4. Balanced Diet: Adopt a diet that is high in whole foods, low in sugar, and supportive of general health in order to combat candida. Stress levels can be positively impacted by proper eating.

5. Herbs and Supplements: Take into account herbs or supplements such as ashwagandha, rhodiola, or magnesium that are proven to relieve stress.

6. Ask for Assistance: Discuss worries or sources of stress with loved ones, friends, or a therapist. Relationships that are supportive can reduce stress.

7. Time Management: Set priorities and organize work to lessen feelings of overburden.

8. Mind-Body Practices: Learn about mind-body techniques that balance both physical and mental well-being, such as acupuncture, tai chi, and qigong.

9. Limit Caffeine and Stimulants: Cut back on caffeine and stimulant consumption as these substances can raise stress and anxiety levels.

10. Healthy Boundaries and Self-Care: Establish boundaries to control stress brought on by relationships, the workplace, or other outside variables. Make self-care activities that make you happy and relaxed a priority.

Sleep, Exercise, and Candida Control

Exercise and getting enough sleep are crucial elements of a healthy lifestyle that can help with Candida control. Both are essential for maintaining overall health and the immune system, which are key components in controlling Candida overgrowth. They support Candida control in the following ways:

Rest:

1. The Immune System: Getting enough sleep is essential for a strong immune system. Getting enough sleep helps immune cells fight off infections, such as Candida overgrowth.

2. Hormonal Balance: Sleep affects how hormones are regulated, which helps to keep the internal environment balanced and prevent the overgrowth of Candida.

3. Stress Reduction: Restful sleep lowers stress, and as a resilient body is more resilient to stress, this can indirectly help promote Candida control.

Workout:

1. Boosts Immunity: Frequent exercise strengthens the immune system, assisting in the fight against illnesses, including Candida overgrowth.

2. De-stressing: Exercise is an effective way to reduce stress, as it lowers stress hormones that can impair immunity and fuel the growth of Candida.

3. Improves Circulation: Better circulation facilitates the evacuation of waste and the supply of nutrients, creating a healthier internal environment that can impede the growth of Candida.

Methods for Using Exercise and Sleep to Control Candida:

1. Make sleep a priority: Try to get 7-9 hours of good sleep every night. To enhance the quality of your sleep, set up a soothing nighttime routine and a regular sleep regimen.

2. Incorporate Frequent Exercise: Work out at a moderate to high level most days of the week. Look for things to do that you enjoy, like swimming, cycling, yoga, or walking.

3. Fuse the Two: Together, maintaining a regular sleep schedule and adding exercise to your daily routine can boost immunity and general health, which will help manage Candida.

4. Balance and Moderation: Steer clear of extreme physical stress or workouts that are too rigorous, as these might weaken the immune system.

Detoxification Techniques

The goal of detoxification treatments is to aid the body's inherent systems for getting rid of waste and poisons. Although there is little scientific data that directly links detoxification techniques to the management of Candida overgrowth, some approaches may help manage Candida overgrowth by indirectly enhancing general health. The following general detoxification methods are some things to think about:

1. A nutritious diet:

 A diet against candida: To support the body's natural detoxification pathways, eat a diet high in whole foods, vegetables, lean proteins, and healthy fats and low in refined carbohydrates and sugars.

2. Aqueous:

Intake of Water: Drink plenty of water to help your kidneys work better and to make it easier for your urine to flush out pollutants.

3. Enhancing Liver Function:

Foods That Support Liver Function: Include foods that boost liver function, such as garlic, onions, beets, cruciferous vegetables (broccoli, cauliflower), and leafy greens.

4. Sweating:

Exercise: Exert yourself to create sweat, which will help the skin flush out toxins.

5. Herbal Teas:

Teas that Detoxify: It's thought that some herbal teas, such as nettle, milk thistle, and dandelion root, aid in liver detoxification.

6. Semi-Annular Fasting:

Times of Fasting: Fasting on occasion or intermittently can help the body's natural detoxification and cellular repair processes.

7. Aiding with Digestive Health: The probiotics indirectly aid in detoxification by fostering a healthy gut flora through the consumption of probiotic-rich meals or supplements.

8. Steam rooms or saunas:

Heat therapy: Sweating in saunas or steam rooms may aid in the elimination of toxins.

9. Minimizing Exposure to Toxins:

Restrict Exposure to Toxins: Reduce your exposure to pollutants in the environment by using natural personal care and cleaning products.

10. Mind-Body Techniques:

De-stressing: Reduce stress by using relaxation methods like yoga, meditation, or deep breathing exercises. This will help with detoxification.

Vital Points to Remember:

Speak with a Professional: See a healthcare provider prior to beginning any detox program, particularly if you are taking medication or have underlying medical conditions.

Gradual Changes: Adopt detoxification techniques gradually to give the body time to acclimate and to prevent significant changes that could lead to stress.

CHAPTER FIVE

NATURAL REMEDIES

Herbal and Homeopathic Solutions

Of course! Herbal and homeopathic therapies are sometimes regarded as supplementary methods for controlling the overgrowth of Candida. Here are a few frequently recommended choices:

Botanical Remedies:

1. Garlic (Allium sativum): raw or supplemented, garlic is known for its antifungal qualities.

2. Origano Oil (Origanum vulgare): Has antifungal qualities due to the presence of chemicals like thymol and carvacrol. It comes in pill or oil form.

3. Grapefruit Seed Extract: Available in liquid or capsule form, this extract has been researched for possible antifungal properties.

4. Caprylic acid (found in coconut oil): a naturally occurring fatty acid with potential antifungal effects. accessible as an add-on.

5. Tabebuia impetiginosa, or dau d'arco, is an herb having antifungal qualities. accessible as a supplement or tea.

Holistic Remedies:

1. Candida albicans (homeopathic remedy): Candida overgrowth symptoms are addressed in homeopathy with this remedy. A homeopath should advise on the precise dilution and application.

2. Sulfur (Homeopathic Remedy): This may be taken into consideration in situations of severe skin eruptions, redness, and itching associated with Candida.

Vital Points to Remember:

Speak with a Professional: Before utilizing herbal or homeopathic medicines, get advice from a trained herbalist, homeopath, or healthcare provider, particularly if you are on medication or have underlying medical issues.

Discernible Reactions: Reactions to homeopathic and herbal medicines can differ from person to person. It's critical to keep an eye out for any negative encounters or reactions.

Standard Treatment Integration: Rather than being stand-alone treatments, these cures are frequently utilized in conjunction with conventional therapies or lifestyle modifications.

Essential Oils for Candida

Of course! Because of their well-known antibacterial qualities, essential oils are occasionally included in natural strategies for controlling Candida overgrowth. The following essential oils are thought to have antifungal qualities:

1. Melaleuca alternifolia, or tea tree oil: Is well-known for having strong antibacterial and antifungal qualities. It is frequently applied topically in diluted form.

2. Oregano Oil (Origanum vulgare): Has antifungal qualities due to the presence of chemicals like thymol and carvacrol. In diluted form, it is applied topically.

3. Clove Oil (Syzygium aromaticum): Eugenol, which has antibacterial and antifungal actions, is present in this oil. In diluted form, it is applied topically.

4. Lavandula angustifolia (Lavender Oil): Lavender oil is recognized for its relaxing benefits, but it also has some antifungal qualities. In aromatherapy, it is frequently utilized.

 5. Cinnamon Bark Oil (Cinnamomum verum): has an antifungal compound called cinnamon aldehyde. It is suitable for topical treatments when diluted.

6. Thyme Oil (Thymus vulgaris): This oil has thymol, which has antifungal properties. In diluted form, it is applied topically.

Vital Points to Remember:

Application and Dilution: Before applying essential oils topically, dilute them appropriately in a carrier oil to prevent allergic reactions or skin irritation.

Fixed Test: Before using a product widely, conduct a patch test on a small area of skin to check for any adverse reactions.

Advise: Before using essential oils, it is best to speak with a medical expert or an aromatherapist, particularly if you have sensitive skin or underlying medical concerns.

Probiotics and Supplements

Probiotics and specific supplements are often seen as components of a comprehensive strategy to maintain gut health and control Candida overgrowth. Here are a few probiotics and vitamins that are frequently used:

Take probiotics.

1. Lactobacillus acidophilus: Often present in yogurt and supplements, this microbe may aid in the restoration of a balanced gut flora.

2. Lactobacillus rhamnosus: well-known for its capacity to uphold intestinal homeostasis and assist immunological activity.

3. Bifidobacterium bifidum: may help improve digestion and regulate the intestinal environment.

4. Saccharomyces boulardii: A probiotic based on yeast that can aid in reestablishing intestinal balance. It's frequently taken either during or after an antibiotic course.

Extra Materials:

1. Caprylic Acid: A naturally occurring fatty acid with antifungal effects that is extracted from coconut oil.

2. Grapefruit Seed Extract: Widely utilized due to possible antifungal properties.

3. Berberine: well-known for its antibacterial qualities and capacity to promote intestinal well-being.

4. Digestive Enzymes: May promote digestion and help break down nutrients, thereby contributing to the preservation of a healthy gut environment.

Vital Points to Remember:

Quality and Dosage: Make sure you choose probiotics and supplements from reliable sources that are of the highest caliber.

Speak with a Professional: Before beginning any new probiotics or supplements, get advice from a qualified dietician or healthcare professional, particularly if you have underlying medical issues or are taking medication.

Personal Reactions: Individuals may react differently to probiotics and vitamins. Keep an eye out for any negative encounters or reactions.

CHAPTER SIX

PRACTICAL TIPS FOR EVERYDAY LIFE

Candida Management at Home

Changing one's lifestyle and using natural therapies to supplement medical treatments are important aspects of managing Candida overgrowth at home. A comprehensive method for controlling Candida overgrowth at home is as follows:

Dietary Modifications:

1. Anti-Candida Diet: Emphasize whole foods, lean proteins, and healthy fats while reducing sugar and refined carbohydrates.

Include foods high in probiotics, low-sugar fruits, and non-starchy veggies.

2. Hydration: Make sure you're getting enough water to help with detoxification and to stay hydrated.

Modifications to Lifestyle:

1. Stress Management: Take part in relaxing pursuits like yoga, meditation, or deep breathing techniques.

2. Sleep and Exercise: To enhance immune system performance and general health, strive for good sleep and frequent exercise.

Organic Solutions:

1. Herbal Solutions: Take into account plants with possible antifungal qualities, such as garlic, oregano oil, or pau d'arco.

2. Probiotics: Restore a healthy gut flora by using probiotics. Select strains and brands that are well known for supporting digestive health.

3. Essential Oils: Certain essential oils, such as oregano or tea tree oil, may be applied topically to treat fungal infections.

Extra Materials:

1. Grapefruit Seed Extract or Caprylic Acid: Take into account products that have antifungal properties, such as grapefruit seed extract or caprylic acid.

2. Digestive Enzymes: Use digestive enzymes to help break down and absorb nutrients.

Self-Care and Hygiene:

1. **Personal Hygiene:** Practice proper hygiene, particularly in warm, humid environments where yeast infections might occur.

2. **Cotton Clothing:** Dress in airy, loose-fitting garments, ideally composed of organic materials like cotton.

Professional Advice

Advise: For individualized guidance, see a herbalist, nutritionist, or healthcare professional.

Review and Sustaining: Keep a close eye on your symptoms and seek additional care if something seems off.

Handling Candida in Social Settings

It may be difficult to navigate social situations while controlling Candida overgrowth, but it is totally doable with a few preparations and adjustments:

1. **Interact with Others:** Let close friends and family members know about your food limitations and medical requirements. This can assist them in comprehending and endorsing your decisions.

2. Arrange in Advance for Get-Togethers: If you're going to events or get-togethers, volunteer to bring a meal that complies with your dietary requirements so you can make sure you have something to eat.

3. Be Aware of Food Selections: Examine menus beforehand or, if you can, inquire with hosts about the meal. Select foods that are vegetable-based, salads without dressings, or grilled meats that meet your dietary restrictions.

4. Avoid temptations: Gently turn down offers that include items that make you feel like you have Candida. If required, include a brief explanation of your dietary limitations.

5. Think About Alcohol and Desserts: Restrict or stay away from alcohol, sweetened drinks, and desserts because they frequently include sugars that might make Candida overgrowth worse.

6. Focus on Social Interaction: Move the emphasis from eating to mingling and interacting with others. Take part in non-eating-related activities, such as walks or other hobbies.

7. Bring Your Own Snacks: To prevent feeling hungry or tempted by non-compliant meals, carry small, portable snacks that meet your dietary restrictions.

8. Remain Upbeat: Remain optimistic about the food you choose to eat. Thank your hosts or friends for making the effort to meet your needs.

9. Educate Without Overwhelming: If appropriate, share facts regarding candida; nevertheless, try not to give too much away.

10. Don't Worry About Mistakes: Don't focus on anything you unintentionally ate that made your symptoms worse. After that, concentrate on getting your diet back on track.

Avoiding Triggers in Daily Routines

Preventing Candida overgrowth in daily life entails making deliberate decisions to reduce exposure to substances that encourage the formation of the infection. These are actions to think about:

Diet

1. Reduce Sugar Intake: Steer clear of processed meals, sugary drinks, and refined sugars, as these can feed Candida.

2. Decrease Carbohydrates: Cut back on refined carbs, which are converted to sugars and found in white bread, spaghetti, and pastries.

3. Control alcohol and coffee. Moderately: Alcohol and too much caffeine can throw off the equilibrium in the gut and encourage the growth of Candida.

Proper wash

1. Maintain good hygiene. To prevent yeast growth, keep skin dry and clean, especially in regions that are prone to wetness.

2. Select Gentle Soaps: To prevent upsetting the skin's natural equilibrium, use moderate, fragrance-free soaps.

Clothes and Textiles:

1. Select Breathable Textiles: Put on airy, loose-fitting clothes, particularly in places where yeast infections are prone to occur.

2. Take off damaged clothes: In order to stop yeast growth in moist settings, immediately remove any damp training clothes or swimwear.

Stress Reduction:

1. Stress Reduction: To enhance general health and immunity, engage in stress-relieving exercises like yoga, meditation, or hobbies.

2. Make Sleep a Priority: To enhance immunity and general wellbeing, make sleep a priority.

Drugs and Medical Conditions:

1. **Antibiotics:** Since antibiotics might alter the gut microbiome, take them sparingly and only as directed by medical professionals.

2. Health disorders: Take good care of any underlying medical disorders you may have, as some erode immunity and make you more vulnerable to Candida overgrowth.

Items for Personal Care:

1. **Steer clear of harmful chemicals:** To prevent upsetting the natural equilibrium of your skin, use mild, natural personal care products.

2. **Restricted Antimicrobial Items:** Overuse of antimicrobial treatments might upset the natural flora on the skin.

Workout:

1. Dress breathableally for your workout: When exercising, choose breathable clothing to avoid moisture accumulation.

2. Post-Workout Shower: To reduce moisture, take a shower and change into dry clothes after working out.

CHAPTER SEVEN

OVERCOMING CHALLENGES

Dealing with Setbacks

Overcoming obstacles while controlling Candida overgrowth is a typical aspect of the process. Here's how to deal with failures well:

1. Remain Upbeat and Patient: Recognize that obstacles are common and a necessary part of the healing process. Remain calm and patient, and keep an optimistic outlook.

2. Reflect and Learn: Determine what could have caused the failure. Was it stress, a nutritional error, or something else entirely? Turn setbacks into teaching moments.

3. Go Back to Your Schedule: Resuming your anti-Candida treatment will help. Maintain the dietary and lifestyle adjustments that were beneficial to you.

4. Pay Attention to Self-Care: When facing difficulties, exercise self-compassion and self-care. Take part in relaxing and stress-relieving activities.

5. Ask for Assistance: Seek advice and encouragement from a support group or a medical practitioner. Ask for help and share your experiences.

6. Reevaluate and Modify: Rethink your strategy. Exist any places that require modification or adjustment? Adapt your strategy in light of your new knowledge.

7. Remain Consistent: Uniformity is essential. Maintain your routine despite difficulties. Long-term gains are often the result of consistent effort.

8. Prevent Overreaction: Steer clear of overreacting to obstacles. Remain composed and refrain from making big decisions that could impede your growth.

9. Monitor Your Development: To keep track of your symptoms, food, and lifestyle, keep a journal. Monitoring makes it easier to see trends and problem areas.

10. Celebrate Small Victories: Honor and commemorate minor victories. Thank you for your efforts; every step you take toward improved health counts.

Emotional and Psychological Impact

It is true that controlling Candida overgrowth can have psychological and emotional effects. Managing symptoms, following dietary guidelines, and receiving long-term treatment can all provide emotional difficulties. Here is how to deal with these elements:

1. Acknowledge Your Feelings: Identify and accept any irritation, tension, or worry you may be experiencing while trying to manage Candida. It's common to experience moments of overwhelm.

2. Ask for Assistance: Discuss your feelings with friends, family, or a therapist. Perspective and relief are two benefits of talking about your emotions.

3. Educate Yourself: Gaining knowledge about Candida overgrowth, its signs, and the course of therapy might help you feel more in control and less anxious.

4. Practice stress reduction: To relax the body and mind, partake in stress-relieving activities like yoga, meditation, or deep breathing exercises.

5. Join Support Groups: Make connections with people who are treating Candida as well. Support groups and online forums can provide direction, empathy, and a shared experience.

6. Focus on What You Can Control: Rather than focusing on the uncontrollable, pay attention to factors that you can influence, such as food decisions and lifestyle modifications.

7. Establish Reasonable Expectations: Have patience as you make progress. Setbacks are common, and healing takes time. Set attainable objectives and acknowledge minor successes.

8. Maintain Balance: Take breaks from controlling Candida by engaging in enjoyable and restorative activities. Don't allow it to rule your life.

9. Exercise self-compassion; treat yourself with kindness. It can be difficult to manage a chronic ailment, so when things get tough, remember to be kind to yourself.

10. Professional Assistance: If anxiety or depression symptoms worsen, think about getting assistance from a therapist or counselor who specializes in treating long-term illnesses.

Seeking Support

When controlling Candida overgrowth, getting help can be very helpful. Here are a few methods to look for assistance:

Medical Service Providers:

1. **Primary Care Physician:** Talk to your primary care physician about your symptoms, available treatments, and any concerns you may have.

2. **Specialists:** Seek advice from professionals with experience treating Candida overgrowth, such as naturopathic physicians, gastroenterologists, or allergists.

Help for Therapy:

1. **Counselors or Therapists**: If taking care of Candida impacts your mental health, get expert assistance. Counselors can help with emotional difficulties and stress management.

2. **Facilities:** Participate in local or online Candida overgrowth support groups. It might be consoling to share experiences and guidance with others.

Dietitians or nutritionists:

1. **Registered Dietitians:** Consult a dietitian who specializes in functional nutrition or gut health. They can help with the creation of customized meal programs for the management of Candida.

Virtual Sources:

1. Forums and Websites: Investigate reliable blogs, websites, and discussion boards devoted to managing candida. Seek out reliable sources for information that is supported by evidence.

2. Online Communities: Become a member of social media pages or groups devoted to Candida overgrowth. Interact with others to provide assistance and exchange experiences.

Family and Friends:

1. Friendly Connections: Discuss your struggles with relatives and friends. Their assistance and comprehension can be quite helpful.

CHAPTER EIGHT

LONG-TERM MAINTENANCE

Sustaining Candida Control

Maintaining Candida control necessitates persistent work and alterations to the lifestyle to avoid relapse. The following are methods to stay in charge:

Eating Patterns:

1. Adhere to the Anti-Candida Diet: Focus on full, nutrient-dense foods and avoid refined carbohydrates, sweets, and yeast-containing foods.

2. Regular Hydration: To aid in detoxing and preserve general health, make sure you are getting enough water.

Modifications to Lifestyle:

1. Stress Management: To enhance immune function, keep up stress-relieving activities like yoga, meditation, or hobbies.

2. Sleep and Exercise: To support general health and immunity, make regular exercise and good sleep a priority.

Sustaining Gut Health:

1. Probiotics: To maintain a healthy gut microbiome, keep consuming foods or supplements high in probiotics.

2. Digestive Support: To help with digestion and nutrient absorption, take into consideration digestive enzymes if necessary.

Self-Care and Hygiene:

1. Maintain Good Hygiene: Keep up your hygiene routines to avoid yeast overgrowth, particularly in places that are prone to moisture.

2. Select Skin-Friendly Items: To keep your skin healthy, use gentle, natural personal care products.

Regularity and Surveillance:

1. Remain Consistent: To avoid a recurrence, stick to the routines and practices that helped control Candida.

2. Consistent Check-ins: To identify any changes early, keep a vigilant eye on your overall health and symptoms.

Professional Advice

1. Regular Follow-ups: To guarantee ongoing development, schedule recurring appointments with medical professionals or specialists.

2. Consultations as Needed: If symptoms return or if new worries emerge, get expert counsel right away.

Assistance Networks:

1. Supportive Community: Keep in touch with forums or support groups for guidance, inspiration, and life lessons.

2. Share Knowledge: You might be able to assist others by imparting your understanding of controlling Candida overgrowth.

Preventing Recurrence

Sustaining a Candida overgrowth requires vigilante care and long-term lifestyle changes. Here's how to reduce the possibility of another incident:

Preserve Dietary Adjustments:

1. Maintain Anti-Candida Diet: Maintain a well-balanced diet that emphasizes whole, nutrient-dense foods and is low in sugars, processed carbohydrates, and yeast-containing foods.

2. Be Aware of Triggers: Restrict intake of recognized triggers, such as processed foods, alcohol, and caffeine, as these may encourage Candida growth.

Encourage Gut Health

1. Probiotics: To keep your gut microbiota healthy, keep eating foods high in probiotics or taking probiotic supplements.

2. Prebiotic Foods: To encourage the growth of advantageous gut flora, include prebiotic-rich foods (such as garlic, onions, and asparagus).

Adopting a Healthier Lifestyle:

1. Stress Management: Continue engaging in stress-reducing activities to promote general wellbeing and a robust immune system.

2. **Regular Exercise:** To strengthen immunity and encourage a healthy interior environment, go moving on a regular basis.

Self-Care and Hygiene:

1. Healthy Personal Habits: Maintain good hygiene habits to avoid yeast overgrowth, particularly in damp places.

2. Skin-Friendly Products: To preserve the health of your skin, use mild, non-irritating personal care products.

Frequent Observation:

1. **Remain Aware of Symptoms*** Keep an eye out for any indications of a relapse or changes in your health, and take quick action if necessary.

2. **Booked Inspections**: To guarantee ongoing health, schedule check-ins or follow-up visits with medical professionals on a regular basis.

Adjust to Specific Needs:

1. **Customize Your Strategy:** Adjust your diet or routine in accordance with your body's reactions and any triggers you find.

2. **Assist When Required:** If you experience any worrisome symptoms or would need advice on how to handle potential triggers, consult a specialist.

Assistance Networks:

1. **Stay Connected:** Participate in forums and support groups going forward to learn from others and stay informed.

2. **Educate people:** Give people access to your expertise and life lessons to help them avoid and control Candida overgrowth.

Healthy Living Beyond Candida

Of course! Beyond Candida, healthy living entails upholding a way of life that promotes general wellbeing. Here are a few crucial areas to concentrate on:

Harmonious Diet:

1. Complete Foods: Stress the importance of eating a diet full of whole, unprocessed foods, such as fruits, vegetables, lean meats, and healthy fats.

2. Moderation: Make moderate dietary choices, indulging in pleasures from time to time but sticking to a mostly healthy diet.

Gut Welfare:

1. Probiotics and prebiotics: To maintain a varied and healthy gut microbiota, keep eating foods high in probiotics and prebiotics.

2. Foods High in Fiber: Include fiber from a variety of sources to help gut flora and digestive health.

Stress Reduction:

1. Stress-Relief Activities: To effectively manage stress levels, partake in stress-relieving activities such as mindfulness, meditation, or hobbies.

2. Work-Life Balance: To promote mental and emotional well-being, strike a balance between your personal, professional, and leisure activities.

Consistent Exercise:

1. Physical Activity: Include regular exercise in your routine to help maintain weight, strengthen your heart, and increase your general vigor.

2. Variety in Workouts: For a well-rounded fitness program, incorporate a variety of cardio, strength training, and flexibility activities.

Restful Sleep:

1. Healthy Sleep Habits: Make quality sleep a priority by keeping a regular sleep schedule and setting up a comfortable sleeping environment.

2. Relaxation Techniques: To decompress and enhance the quality of your sleep, practice relaxation techniques before going to bed.

Be Hydrated:

1. Sufficient Water Intake: Continue to drink enough water throughout the day to keep well-hydrated.

2. Herbal Infusions: For extra health benefits and hydration, try infused water or herbal teas.

Health Preventive Measures:

1. Regular Check-Ups: To keep an eye on general health, schedule regular screenings and check-ups.

2. Health Awareness: To preserve healthiness, keep up to date on medical issues and precautions.

Intentional Living:

1. Mindfulness Practices: To improve concentration and mental clarity, practice mindfulness through yoga, deep breathing techniques, or mindfulness meditation.

2. Gratitude and Positivity: To promote mental and emotional well-being, engage in acts of gratitude and positive thinking.

CONCLUSION

Of course! Controlling Candida overgrowth necessitates a multimodal strategy that includes dietary modifications, lifestyle tweaks, and ongoing attention to detail. Every action helps lessen the effects of Candida, from realizing its origin to putting dietary changes into practice, managing stress, and consulting a professional.

Being knowledgeable about Candida and its triggers is the first step toward making wise decisions. A better internal environment can be supported by following an anti-Candida diet high in whole foods and low in sugar and refined carbohydrates. When combined with stress management methods, physical activity, and sufficient rest, these alterations in lifestyle strengthen the body's defenses against Candida overgrowth.

Probiotics, good hygiene, and consulting a specialist guarantee a well-rounded approach. The emotional toll that controlling Candida takes is recognized, and emphasis is placed on finding support systems and preserving mental health along the way.

Sustained efforts are necessary to prevent recurrence, including maintaining gut health according to individualized demands and maintaining regular dietary practices. Beyond managing Candida, the holistic approach promotes healthy lifestyle habits that include exercise, stress reduction, diet, and preventative healthcare.

In summary, managing Candida overgrowth necessitates commitment, endurance, and a comprehensive approach. One can effectively manage Candida by incorporating these tactics into daily life and maintaining healthy behaviors, which will support general health and vitality even in the absence of Candida. Remember, living a bright, well-balanced life is just as important as managing Candida.

www.ingramcontent.com/pod-product-compliance
Lightning Source LLC
Chambersburg PA
CBHW071102260726
48661CB00006B/2404